# WHOLE

# BODY RESET

# FOR SENIORS

*Simple and Easy Weight Loss Plan
with Healthy Meal Recipes and
Morning Exercises to Boost
Metabolism and Live Healthier*

**Gina Stephens**

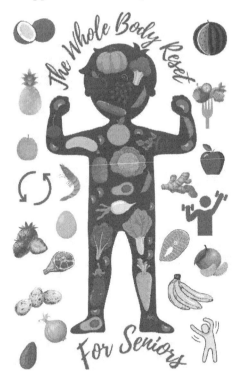

*A better health, a better you!*

# CONTENTS

# INTRODUCTION

As we age, maintaining a healthy weight and nourishing our bodies becomes increasingly important. With each passing decade, our metabolisms tend to slow down, making it more challenging to shed excess pounds and maintain a healthy lifestyle. That's why I felt compelled to write the "Whole Body Reset for Seniors."

After witnessing the struggles that many seniors face when it comes to weight management, I realized the need for a comprehensive resource tailored specifically to their unique needs and challenges. This book is a result of my deep commitment to promoting the well-being of seniors by providing them with practical tools and delicious recipes to support their weight loss journey. It focuses on nourishing the body, boosting energy levels, and enhancing overall health.

The recipes in this book are carefully designed to meet the nutritional requirements of seniors while catering to their taste preferences. They are delicious, satisfying, and easy to prepare, making it convenient for seniors to adopt healthier eating habits without feeling overwhelmed or deprived.

Additionally, this book provides practical tips, meal plans, and guidance on portion control, mindful eating, and maintaining an active lifestyle. I firmly believe that age should never be a barrier to achieving optimal health and well-being. With the "Whole Body Reset for Seniors," I hope to empower seniors to take control of their health, embrace positive changes, and embark on a transformative weight loss journey that will not only help them shed unwanted pounds but also improve their overall quality of life.

So, whether you're a senior looking to shed a few extra pounds, boost your energy levels, or simply adopt a healthier lifestyle, this book is designed with you in mind. Together, let's embark on a path of rejuvenation, vitality, and a whole-body reset that will enable you to live your best life well into your golden years.

# 5 PHASES OF RESETTING

Beginning a weight loss journey can be a positive step towards better health and well-being for seniors. Here are the 5 phases to initiate and maintain a whole body reset routine for weight loss:

**Phase 1: Setting Clear Goals and Planning**

**Consult with a Healthcare Professional:** Before embarking on any weight loss journey, seniors need to consult with a healthcare professional to ensure their safety and well-being. They can provide guidance tailored to individual health conditions and offer recommendations for a unique whole body reset weight loss strategy.

**Define Realistic Goals:** Set achievable and realistic weight loss goals. Seniors should focus on sustainable weight loss rather than rapid results, aiming for a gradual and steady reduction in weight.

**Create a Personalized Plan:** Develop a personalized weight loss plan that takes into account the specific needs and preferences of seniors. Consider factors such as dietary requirements, physical limitations, and any medical conditions.

**Phase 2: Nutrition and Dietary Changes**

**Balanced and Nutrient-Dense Diet:** Seniors should adopt a balanced and nutrient-dense diet that includes a variety of fruits, vegetables, whole grains, lean proteins, and healthy fats. Limit your intake of processed foods, sweet snacks, and drinks.

**Portion Control:** Encourage seniors to practice portion control and mindful eating. This involves being aware of portion sizes and eating until satisfied, rather than overeating.

**Hydration:** Drinking an adequate amount of water is crucial for overall health and weight loss. Seniors should aim to drink at least 8 cups (64 ounces) of water per day unless advised otherwise by a healthcare professional.

**Phase 3: Physical Activity and Exercise**

**Engage in low-impact exercises suitable for seniors:** It helps burn calories, strengthen muscles, and improve cardiovascular health without putting excessive strain on joints.

**Strength Training:** Incorporate strength training exercises into the fitness routine to improve muscle mass and metabolism.

**Flexibility and Balance Exercises:** These activities can improve mobility, reduce the risk of falls, and enhance overall well-being.

Check out the varieties of exercise ideas suitable for seniors in the exercise section of this book.

## Phase 4: Lifestyle Changes

**Quality Sleep:** Encourage seniors to establish a consistent sleep schedule and prioritize getting quality sleep. Aim for 7-8 hours of uninterrupted sleep per night to support weight loss efforts.

**Stress Management:** Help seniors adopt stress management techniques, such as meditation, deep breathing exercises, or engaging in hobbies they enjoy. High-stress levels can contribute to weight gain, so managing stress is crucial for a successful weight loss journey.

**Social Support:** Foster a supportive environment by encouraging seniors to engage in social activities. Having a support system can provide motivation, accountability, and encouragement throughout the weight loss process.

**Phase 5: Monitoring and Adjusting**

**Regular Monitoring:** Regularly monitor progress by tracking weight, measurements, and food intake. Keep a journal or use digital tools to record these details, making it easier to identify patterns and make necessary adjustments.

**Seek Professional Support:** If seniors encounter challenges or feel stuck in their weight loss journey, they should consider seeking support from professionals, such as dietitians, nutritionists, or personal trainers, who specialize in senior health and weight management.

**Adapt and Modify:** Continuously assess and modify the weight loss strategy as needed. As seniors progress, they may need to adjust their exercise routine, and meal plan, or set new goals to maintain their momentum and continue making progress.

# BEST EXERCISES FOR SENIORS

Losing weight is beneficial for individuals of all ages, including seniors. Engaging in regular exercise not only aids in weight management but also promotes overall health and well-being. For seniors, it's important to focus on exercises that are low-impact, gentle on the joints, and cater to their specific needs and abilities. Here are some excellent exercises that seniors can incorporate into their fitness routine to promote weight loss:

**Chair Yoga**

Chair yoga is a modified form of traditional yoga that can be performed while seated on a chair. It involves gentle stretches, breathing exercises, and meditation. Chair yoga improves flexibility, strengthens muscles, and promotes relaxation.

Example: Seated spinal twist - Sit tall in a chair, place your left hand on the outside of your right knee, and gently twist your upper body to the right. Repeat on the opposite side after holding for a few breaths. In addition to the seated spinal twist, chair yoga includes various other poses and stretches that can be done while sitting on a chair.

These may include seated forward folds, gentle twists, side stretches, and leg stretches.

**Marching**

Marching is a simple and effective aerobic exercise that can be done in place. It raises the heart rate, burns calories, and strengthens the leg muscles.

Example: Stand tall with feet hip-width apart and march in place, lifting your knees as high as comfortable. Swing your arms naturally with the rhythm of the march. While marching in place, you can vary the intensity and difficulty by lifting your knees higher or incorporating arm movements. You can also add variations like knee lifts with a twist or alternating knee lifts to engage your core muscles.

**Step Jacks**

Step jacks are a low-impact variation of jumping jacks. They provide a cardiovascular workout while reducing stress on the joints.

Example: Stand with feet together and step your right foot out to the side, simultaneously raising both arms overhead. Follow the same steps on the other side, then go back to your starting point. It can be modified by reducing the range of motion or performing the movements at a slower pace.

**Quick Feet**

Quick feet exercises are a fun way to improve cardiovascular fitness and burn calories. They involve fast footwork and can be done at a moderate intensity level.

Example: Stand with feet hip-width apart and rapidly tap your feet on the floor, lifting them just a few inches off the ground. As you become more comfortable, speed up.

**Alternating Reach Knee Lift**

This exercise targets the core, improves balance, and engages the leg muscles. It can be done using a chair for support if needed.

Example: Stand tall with feet hip-width apart. Lift your right knee toward your chest while simultaneously reaching your left arm overhead. Repeat on the other side, lowering the arm and leg.

**Pilates**

Pilates is a low-impact training technique that emphasizes core strength, flexibility, and posture. It can help seniors build lean muscle, improve balance, and enhance body awareness.

Example: Perform the Pilates "Leg Circle" exercise by lying on your back, extending one leg toward the ceiling, and making controlled circles with your leg. Repeat with the other leg. Apart from leg circles, other common Pilates exercises for seniors include pelvic tilts, bridging, leg slides, and arm circles.

**Water Aerobics**

Water aerobics provides a low-impact, joint-friendly workout by utilizing the resistance of water. It improves cardiovascular fitness, strength, and flexibility.

Example: Perform a water jogging exercise by moving through the water with a jogging motion, lifting your knees, and swinging your arms as if you were jogging on land. Other examples include leg kicks, arm movements, and resistance exercises using water dumbbells or noodles.

**Dumbbell Strength Training**

Strength training with dumbbells helps build lean muscle mass, increase metabolism, and promote weight loss. It is essential for maintaining muscle strength as we age.

Example: Perform bicep curls by holding dumbbells in each hand, palms facing forward. Curl the weights up towards your shoulders while keeping your elbows tight to your body. Other examples include overhead presses, lateral raises, triceps extensions, and squats with weights.

## Bodyweight Workouts

Bodyweight exercises use your body as resistance and require no additional equipment. They can enhance your flexibility, strength, and stamina. Example: Perform squats by standing with feet hip-width apart, bending your knees, and lowering your body as if you were sitting back in a chair. Return to the starting position and repeat. Other examples to try out include lunges, modified push-ups against a wall or countertop, standing calf raises, and chair dips.

## Walking

Walking is a convenient, low-impact workout that can be done anywhere. It improves cardiovascular health, strengthens leg muscles, and aids in weight management. Example: Take brisk walks in your neighborhood or on a treadmill for at least 30 minutes a day. Gradually increase your pace and distance as you become more comfortable.

## Resistance Band Workouts

Resistance bands offer a convenient and portable way to incorporate strength training into your routine. They provide resistance to help build muscle and burn calories.

Example: Perform seated rows by sitting on a chair with legs extended, loop the resistance band around your feet, and grasp the band with both hands. Squeeze your shoulder blades together as you pull the band towards your body. Besides seated rows, you can perform exercises like bicep curls, lateral raises, triceps extensions, squats with resistance bands around your thighs, and seated leg presses.

Exercises be avoided for seniors over the age of 65:

- Jumping jacks
- High-impact aerobics
- Heavy weightlifting
- Overhead shoulder press
- Military press
- Trampolining
- Dancing with jarring movements
- Fall-risk exercises
- High-intensity interval training (HIIT)
- Advanced yoga poses
- Exercises on unstable surfaces (e.g., stability ball)
- Deep side bends
- Full sit-ups
- Exercises involving rapid spinal rotations

Remember to start slowly and consult with a healthcare professional before beginning any new exercise program, especially if you have pre-existing medical conditions. Additionally, listen to your body and adjust the intensity and duration of exercises according to your comfort level. Regular physical activity, combined with a healthy diet, will support weight loss efforts and contribute to improved overall health for seniors.

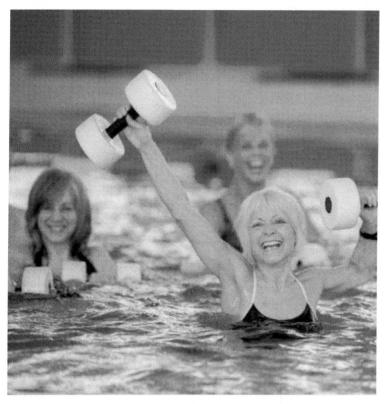

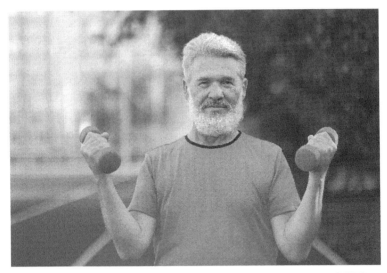

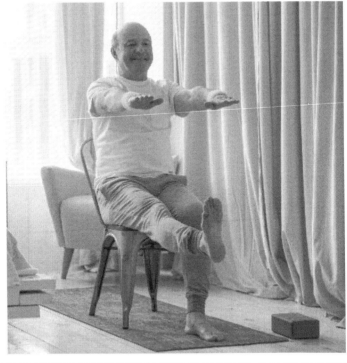

# MINDFULNESS PRACTICES

Mindfulness practices can be immensely beneficial for seniors who are embarking on a whole body reset journey, aiming to develop a positive relationship with food, manage emotional eating, and reduce stress levels. Here are some mindfulness techniques that can support these goals:

**Mindful Eating**

Encourages seniors to practice mindful eating by paying attention to their food and the act of eating. Suggest the following steps:

- **Engage their senses:** This encourages them to notice the colors, textures, and aromas of their food.

- **Slow down:** Advises seniors to eat slowly, savoring each bite and chewing thoroughly.

- **Listen to their body:** Encourages seniors to tune in to their body's hunger and fullness cues, eating until satisfied, not overly full.

- **Non-judgmental awareness:** Teaches seniors to observe their thoughts and emotions without judgment or criticism.

## Body Scan Meditation

Guides seniors through a body scan meditation to cultivate awareness of their physical sensations. Instruct them to:

- **Find a comfortable position:** Encourages seniors to lie down or sit in a relaxed posture.

- **Bring attention to their body:** Guides seniors to gradually shift their focus from head to toe, noticing any areas of tension or discomfort.

- **Release tension:** Instructs seniors to breathe into areas of tension and consciously release it with each exhale.

- **Cultivate gratitude:** Encourages seniors to express gratitude for their body's abilities and to approach their weight loss journey with self-compassion.

## Breath Awareness

Helps seniors develop a mindfulness practice centered around their breath. They can:

- **Find a quiet space:** Advises them to sit comfortably and close their eyes.

- **Focus on the breath:** Instructs them to observe the natural rhythm of their breath, noticing the sensation of the breath entering and leaving the body.

- **Return to the breath:** When the mind wanders, this reminds them to gently bring their attention back to the breath without judgment.
- **Use the breath as an anchor:** Encourages them to use the breath as an anchor to ground themselves in the present moment, especially during stressful or emotional eating situations.

**Daily Gratitude Practice**

- Encourages seniors to incorporate a daily gratitude practice to shift their focus towards positivity and reduce stress levels. They can:
- **Keep a gratitude journal:** Suggests seniors write down three things they are grateful for each day.
- **Reflect on positive moments:** Advises them to take a few moments each day to recall positive experiences and appreciate the simple pleasures in life.
- **Express gratitude to others:** Encourages them to express gratitude to loved ones, caregivers, or friends, fostering positive relationships and social connections.

**Mindful Movement:**

Recommends seniors engage in mindful movement practices such as yoga, tai chi, or gentle stretching exercises. These activities can help them:

- **Cultivate body awareness:** Assists seniors in connecting with their bodies and their physical sensations.

- **Reduce stress and tension:** Supports them in releasing stress and promoting relaxation.

- **Enhance mindfulness:** Guides them to focus on their breath and the present moment during the practice.

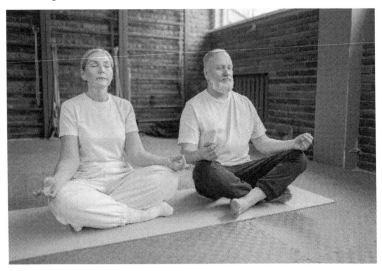

# FOOD RULES

## Foods to Eat

When embarking on a whole body reset journey, it's important for seniors to focus on consuming a well-balanced diet that promotes weight loss and supports overall health. Here is a list of foods that can be beneficial for seniors in their weight loss journey:

**Lean Proteins:**

- Skinless chicken or turkey breast
- Fish like trout, salmon, or tuna
- Eggs
- Greek yogurt
- Beans and legumes (e.g., lentils, chickpeas, black beans)

**Fiber-Rich Fruits and Vegetables:**

- Berries (strawberries, blueberries, raspberries)
- Leafy greens (spinach, kale, lettuce)
- Cruciferous vegetables (broccoli, cauliflower, Brussels sprouts)
- Citrus fruits (oranges, grapefruits)
- Apples

- Avocado
- Carrots

**Whole Grains:**

- Quinoa
- Brown rice
- Oats
- Whole wheat bread or pasta
- Barley

**Healthy Fats:**

- Olive oil
- Nuts and seeds (almonds, walnuts, chia seeds)
- Nut butter (peanut butter, almond butter)
- Flaxseeds
- Fatty fish (salmon, mackerel, sardines)

**Dairy or Dairy Alternatives:**

- Low-fat milk or yogurt
- Cottage cheese
- Unsweetened almond milk or soy milk

**Hydration:**

- Water
- Herbal teas
- Infused water (with fruits or herbs)

**Herbs and Spices:**

- Turmeric
- Cinnamon
- Ginger
- Garlic
- Basil
- Rosemary
- Cayenne pepper

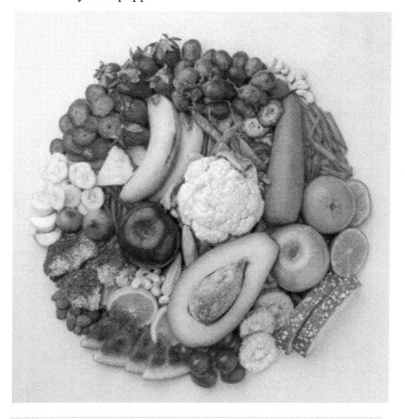

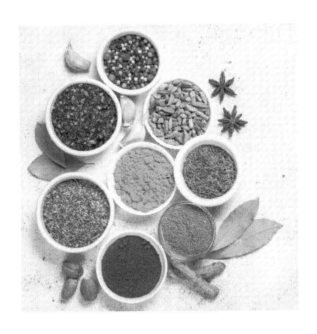

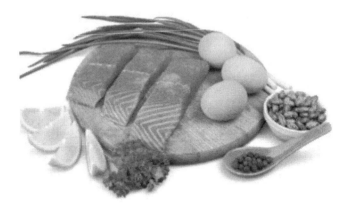

# Foods to Avoid

**Processed Foods:**

- Packaged snacks,
- Frozen meals
- Fast food

Typically high in unhealthy fats, added sugars, and sodium.

**Sugary Drinks:**

- Sodas
- Fruit juices
- Sweetened beverages

**Sweets and Desserts:**

- Cakes, cookies
- Candies
- Other sugary treats

**High-Fat Dairy Products:**

- Full-fat milk
- Cheese
- Ice cream

They can be high in saturated fats.

**Fried Foods:**

- French fries
- Fried chicken
- Tempura

They are often high in unhealthy fat.

**Highly Processed Meats:**

- Sausages
- Bacon
- Deli meats

They contain high levels of sodium, unhealthy fats, and preservatives.

**White Bread and Pasta:**

These refined grains have minimal nutritional value and can cause blood sugar spikes.

**Sugary Cereals:**

Many breakfast cereals are loaded with added sugars and lack essential nutrients.

**Salty Snacks:**

- Chips
- Pretzels
- Salted nuts

They are often high in sodium, which can contribute to high blood pressure and fluid retention.

**Artificial Sweeteners:**

While low in calories, artificial sweeteners can disrupt the body's natural response to sugar and may increase cravings for sweet foods.

# 15-DAY BODY RESET MEAL PLAN

## Day 1:

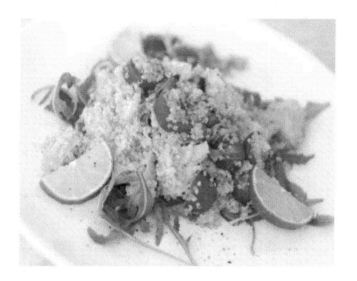

## Breakfast - Green Power Smoothie
**Ingredients:**

- 1 cup spinach
- 1 ripe banana
- ½ cucumber
- 1 tablespoon chia seeds
- 1 cup almond milk (unsweetened)

**Preparation:**

- In a blender, put all the ingredients and blend thoroughly until smooth.
- Serve chilled.

## Lunch - Quinoa Salad

**Ingredients:**

- 1 cup cooked quinoa
- ½ cup cherry tomatoes, halved
- ½ cup diced cucumber
- ¼ cup chopped red onion
- 2 tablespoons chopped fresh parsley
- Juice of 1 lemon
- 1 tablespoon olive oil
- Salt and pepper to taste

**Preparation:**

- In a large bowl, combine quinoa, cherry tomatoes, cucumber, red onion, and parsley.
- Whisk together lemon juice, olive oil, salt, and pepper in a small bowl.
- Toss the quinoa salad with the dressing to combine.
- Serve chilled.

# Dinner - Baked Salmon with Roasted Vegetables

**Ingredients:**

- 1 salmon fillet
- 1 tablespoon olive oil
- 1 teaspoon dried dill
- Salt and pepper to taste
- 1 cup broccoli florets
- 1 cup cauliflower florets
- 1 cup sliced bell peppers
- 1 tablespoon balsamic vinegar

**Preparation:**

- Preheat the oven to 375°F (190°C).
- Line a baking sheet with parchment paper and place the salmon fillet on top.
- Drizzle the salmon with olive oil and sprinkle with dried dill, salt, and pepper.
- In a separate bowl, toss the broccoli florets, cauliflower florets, and bell peppers with olive oil, salt, and pepper.
- On the baking sheet, arrange the vegetables around the salmon.
- Drizzle the vegetables with balsamic vinegar.

- Bake the salmon and vegetables for 15 to 20 mins, or until it is cooked through.
- Serve hot.

## Day 2:

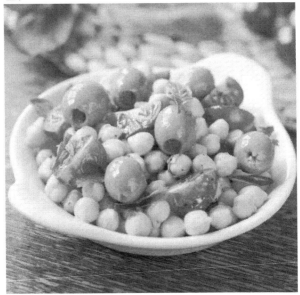

## Breakfast - Berry Blast Smoothie
**Ingredients:**

- 1 cup of straw-blue-raspberries
- 1 ripe banana
- 1 cup unsweetened Greek yogurt
- 1 tablespoon honey (optional)
- ½ cup almond milk (unsweetened)

**Preparation:**

- In a blender, put all the ingredients and blend thoroughly until smooth.
- For additional sweetness, you may add honey if you wish.
- Serve chilled.

# Lunch - Mediterranean Chickpea Salad

**Ingredients:**

- 1 can chickpeas, rinsed and drained
- ½ cup cherry tomatoes, halved
- ½ cup diced cucumber
- ¼ cup sliced Kalamata olives
- 2 tablespoons crumbled feta cheese
- 2 tablespoons chopped fresh parsley
- Juice of 1 lemon
- 1 tablespoon olive oil
- Salt and pepper to taste

**Preparation:**

- Mix chickpeas with the Kalamata olives, cucumber, feta cheese, parsley, and cherry tomatoes in a large bowl.
- Whisk together the lemon juice, olive oil, salt, and pepper in a small bowl.

- Toss the chickpea salad in the dressing to mix.
- Serve chilled.

# Dinner - Grilled Chicken with Steamed Asparagus

**Ingredients:**

- 1 chicken breast
- 1 tablespoon olive oil
- 1 teaspoon dried oregano
- Salt and pepper to taste
- 1 bunch asparagus, trimmed
- Lemon wedges for serving

**Preparation:**

- Preheat the grill to medium-high heat.
- Rub the chicken breast with olive oil, dried oregano, salt, and pepper.
- On the grill, place the chicken and grill for 6 to 8 mins on each side or until done.
- Meanwhile, steam the asparagus until tender.
- Serve the grilled chicken with steamed asparagus and lemon wedges.
- Enjoy!

**Day 3:**

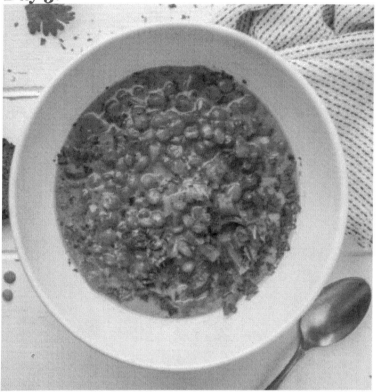

## Breakfast - Tropical Paradise Smoothie
**Ingredients:**

- 1 cup chopped pineapple
- ½ ripe mango, peeled and diced
- ½ cup coconut milk
- 1 tablespoon flaxseeds
- ½ cup orange juice

**Preparation:**

- In a blender, put all the ingredients and blend thoroughly until smooth.
- Serve chilled.

# Lunch - Spinach and Feta Stuffed Chicken Breast

**Ingredients:**

- 1 chicken breast
- 1 cup fresh spinach leaves
- 2 tablespoons crumbled feta cheese
- Salt and pepper to taste
- 1 tablespoon olive oil

**Preparation:**

- Preheat the oven to 400°F (200°C).
- Slice the chicken breast horizontally, creating a pocket.
- Stuff the pocket with fresh spinach leaves and crumbled feta cheese.
- Add salt and pepper to season the chicken breast.
- Over medium-high heat in an oven-safe skillet, heat the olive oil.
- The chicken breast should be seared until golden brown on both sides.

- Move the skillet to the oven and bake for 15 to 20 mins
- Serve hot.

## Dinner - Lentil Vegetable Soup

**Ingredients:**

- 1 cup dried lentils, rinsed
- 1 onion, chopped
- 2 carrots, diced
- 2 celery stalks, diced
- 2 garlic cloves, minced
- 4 cups vegetable broth
- 1 teaspoon dried thyme
- Salt and pepper to taste
- Fresh parsley for garnish

**Preparation:**

- Sauté the onion, celery, carrots, and garlic in a large pot until softened.
- Add lentils, vegetable broth, dried thyme, salt, and pepper to the pot.
- Bring the soup to a boil, then reduce heat and simmer for 20-25 minutes or until the lentils are tender.
- Adjust seasoning if needed.

- Garnish with fresh parsley.
- Serve hot.

## Day 4:

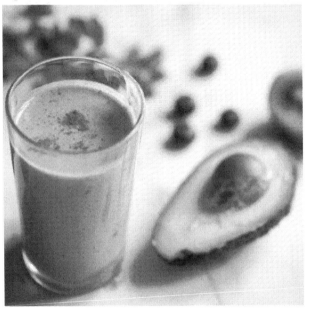

## Breakfast - Green Detox Smoothie
**Ingredients:**

- 1 cup kale leaves
- 1 ripe pear, cored and diced
- ½ avocado
- 1 tablespoon fresh ginger, grated
- 1 tablespoon lemon juice
- 1 cup coconut water

**Preparation:**

- In a blender, put all the ingredients and blend thoroughly until smooth.
- Serve chilled.

## Lunch - Caprese Salad

**Ingredients:**

- 1 large tomato, sliced
- 4 ounces fresh mozzarella cheese, sliced
- ½ cup fresh basil leaves
- 1 tablespoon balsamic glaze
- 1 tablespoon extra-virgin olive oil
- Salt and pepper to taste

**Preparation:**

- Arrange tomato slices, mozzarella slices, and basil leaves on a plate.
- Use balsamic glaze and olive oil to drizzle the salad.
- Season with salt and pepper.
- Serve at room temperature.

## Dinner - Shrimp Stir-Fry with Brown Rice

**Ingredients:**

- 8 ounces shrimp, peeled and deveined
- 1 tablespoon low-sodium soy sauce

- 1 tablespoon hoisin sauce
- 1 tablespoon sesame oil
- 1 tablespoon olive oil
- 1 garlic clove, minced
- 1 teaspoon grated ginger
- 1 cup mixed vegetables (broccoli, bell peppers, carrots)
- 1 cup cooked brown rice

**Preparation:**

- In a bowl, marinate the shrimp with soy sauce and hoisin sauce for 10 minutes.
- Over medium-high heat, in a large skillet or wok heat the sesame oil and olive oil.
- Add garlic and ginger to the skillet and stir-fry for 1 minute.
- Add the marinated shrimp and stir-fry until pink and cooked through.
- Add the mixed vegetables and stir-fry for an additional 2-3 minutes.
- Over the cooked brown rice, serve the shrimp stir-fry.
- Enjoy!

# Day 5:

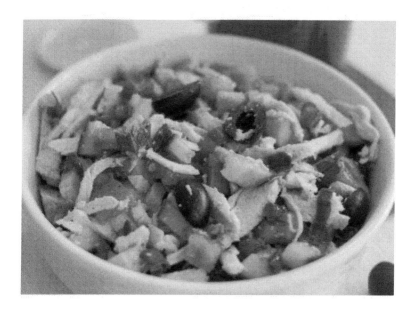

## Breakfast - Banana Nut Smoothie
**Ingredients:**

- 1 ripe banana
- 2 tablespoons almond butter
- 1 cup almond milk (unsweetened)
- 1 tablespoon honey (optional)
- 1 tablespoon crushed walnuts

**Preparation:**

- Blend the ripe banana, almond butter, almond milk, and honey (if desired) until smooth.
- Top with crushed walnuts.
- Serve chilled.

## Lunch - Greek Salad with Grilled Chicken

**Ingredients:**

- 1 chicken breast, grilled and sliced
- 2 cups mixed salad greens
- ¼ cup sliced red onion
- ½ cup cherry tomatoes, halved
- ½ cup diced cucumber
- ¼ cup Kalamata olives
- 2 tablespoons crumbled feta cheese
- 1 tablespoon extra-virgin olive oil
- Juice of 1 lemon
- Salt and pepper to taste

**Preparation:**

- In a large bowl, combine mixed salad greens, red onion, cherry tomatoes, cucumber, Kalamata olives, and crumbled feta cheese.
- Drizzle with olive oil and lemon juice.

- Season with salt and pepper.
- Top with grilled chicken slices.
- Serve chilled.

## Dinner - Lemon-Garlic Sauce with Baked Cod

**Ingredients:**

- 1 cod fillet
- 1 tablespoon olive oil
- Juice of 1 lemon
- 2 garlic cloves, minced
- Salt and pepper to taste
- Fresh parsley for garnish

**Preparation:**

- Preheat the oven to 375°F (190°C).
- Line a baking sheet with parchment paper and place the cod fillet on top.
- Use the olive oil and lemon juice to drizzle the cod.
- Sprinkle minced garlic, salt, and pepper over the cod.
- Bake the cod for 15-20 mins, or until it flakes easily.
- Garnish with fresh parsley.
- Serve hot.

# Day 6:

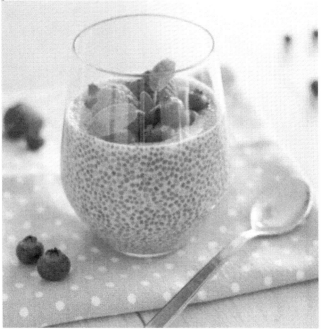

## Breakfast - Mixed Berry Chia Pudding

**Ingredients:**

- 1 cup straw-blue-raspberries
- 2 tablespoons chia seeds
- 1 cup almond milk (unsweetened)
- 1 tablespoon honey (optional)
- Fresh mint leaves for garnish

**Preparation:**

- In a blender, put all the mixed berries and blend thoroughly until smooth.

- Mix the chia seeds and almond milk in a bowl.
- Stir in the blended mixed berries and honey (if desired).
- To make the mixture thicken, place in the refrigerator for at least 2 hours or overnight.
- Garnish with fresh mint leaves.
- Serve chilled.

## Lunch - Quinoa Stuffed Bell Peppers
**Ingredients:**

- 2 bell peppers, halved and seeds removed
- 1 cup cooked quinoa
- ½ cup black beans rinsed and drained
- ½ cup corn kernels
- ½ cup diced tomatoes
- ½ cup diced red onion
- ¼ cup chopped fresh cilantro
- 1 tablespoon lime juice
- 1 teaspoon ground cumin
- Salt and pepper to taste

**Preparation:**

- Preheat the oven to 375°F (190°C).
- Place the bell pepper halves on a baking sheet lined with parchment paper.

- In a large bowl, combine cooked quinoa, black beans, corn kernels, diced tomatoes, red onion, cilantro, lime juice, ground cumin, salt, and pepper.
- Place a spoonful of the quinoa mixture inside each bell pepper half.
- Bake for 20-25 minutes or until the bell peppers are tender and the filling is heated through.
- Serve hot.

## Dinner - Grilled Vegetable Skewers with Tofu

**Ingredients:**

- 8 ounces firm cut into cubes, tofu
- 1 zucchini, sliced
- 1 yellow squash, sliced
- 1 red onion, cut into chunks
- 1 bell pepper, cut into chunks
- 8 cherry tomatoes
- 2 tablespoons olive oil
- 1 tablespoon balsamic vinegar
- 1 teaspoon dried Italian herb
- Salt and pepper to taste

**Preparation:**

- Preheat the grill to medium-high heat.

- Thread tofu cubes, zucchini slices, yellow squash slices, red onion chunks, bell pepper chunks, and cherry tomatoes onto skewers.
- In a small bowl, whisk together olive oil, balsamic vinegar, dried Italian herbs, salt, and pepper.
- Brush the olive oil mixture on the vegetable skewers.
- Grill the skewers for 8-10 minutes, turning occasionally, or until the vegetables are tender and lightly charred.
- Serve hot.

**Day 7:**

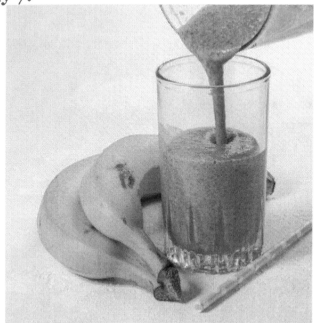

# Breakfast - Spinach and Banana Smoothie

**Ingredients:**

- 1 cup spinach
- 1 ripe banana
- ½ cup unsweetened Greek yogurt
- 1 tablespoon almond butter
- 1 cup almond milk (unsweetened)
- 1 tablespoon honey (optional)

**Preparation:**

- In a blender, put all the ingredients and blend thoroughly until smooth.
- For additional sweetness, add honey if you wish.
- Serve chilled.

## Lunch - Lentil Spinach Salad

**Ingredients:**

- 1 cup cooked lentils
- 2 cups fresh spinach leaves
- ¼ cup diced red onion
- ½ cup diced cucumber
- ¼ cup crumbled goat cheese
- 2 tablespoons chopped fresh dill
- Juice of 1 lemon

- 1 tablespoon olive oil
- Salt and pepper to taste

**Preparation:**

- In a large bowl, combine cooked lentils, spinach leaves, red onion, cucumber, goat cheese, and fresh dill.
- Mix the lemon juice, olive oil, salt, and pepper in a small bowl.
- Toss the lentil spinach salad with the dressing to mix.
- Serve chilled.

# Dinner - Roasted Brussels Sprouts and Baked Chicken Thighs

**Ingredients:**

- 2 chicken thighs
- 1 tablespoon olive oil
- 1 teaspoon smoked paprika
- 1 teaspoon garlic powder
- Salt and pepper to taste
- 1 cup of trimmed and halved Brussels sprouts
- 1 tablespoon balsamic vinegar

**Preparation:**

- Preheat the oven to 375°F (190°C).

- On a baking sheet lined with parchment paper, place the chicken thighs.
- Drizzle the chicken with olive oil and sprinkle with smoked paprika, garlic powder, salt, and pepper.
- In a separate bowl, toss the Brussels sprouts with olive oil, salt, and pepper.
- Arrange the Brussels sprouts around the chicken on the baking sheet.
- Use the balsamic vinegar to drizzle the Brussels sprouts.
- Bake for 25-30 minutes or until the chicken is cooked through and the Brussels sprouts are tender.
- Serve hot.

## Day 8:

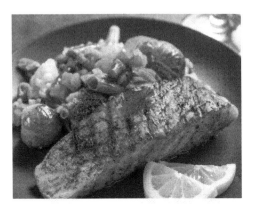

# Breakfast - Berry Blast Smoothie Bowl

**Ingredients:**

- 1 cup frozen straw-blue-raspberries
- 1 ripe banana
- ½ cup unsweetened Greek yogurt
- ¼ cup almond milk (unsweetened)
- 1 tablespoon honey (optional)

**Toppings:**

- Chia seeds
- Granola
- Shredded coconut
- Sliced banana

**Preparation:**

- In a blender, blend the frozen mixed berries, ripe banana, Greek yogurt, almond milk, and honey (if desired) until smooth.
- Pour the smoothie into a bowl.
- Decorate with the toppings.
- Serve chilled.

# Lunch - Mediterranean Chickpea Salad

**Ingredients:**

- 1 can chickpeas, rinsed and drained
- ½ cup diced cucumber

- ½ cup diced tomatoes
- ¼ cup diced red onion
- ¼ cup chopped Kalamata olives
- ¼ cup crumbled feta cheese
- 2 tablespoons chopped fresh parsley
- Juice of 1 lemon
- 1 tablespoon extra-virgin olive oil
- Salt and pepper to taste

**Preparation:**

- In a large bowl, combine chickpeas, cucumber, tomatoes, red onion, Kalamata olives, feta cheese, and fresh parsley.
- Whisk together lemon juice, olive oil, salt, and pepper in a small bowl.
- Toss the chickpea salad in the dressing to mix.
- Serve chilled.

# Dinner - Grilled Salmon with Roasted Vegetables

**Ingredients:**

- 1 salmon fillet
- 1 tablespoon olive oil
- Juice of 1 lemon
- 1 teaspoon dried dill

- Salt and pepper to taste
- 1 cup mixed vegetables (broccoli, bell peppers, carrots)
- 1 tablespoon balsamic vinegar

**Preparation:**

- Preheat the grill to medium-high heat.
- On a piece of aluminum foil, arrange the salmon fillet.
- Drizzle the salmon with olive oil and lemon juice.
- Sprinkle dried dill, salt, and pepper over the salmon.
- Fold the aluminum foil to create a packet around the salmon.
- Grill the salmon packet for 10-12 minutes or until the salmon is cooked through.
- In the meantime, toss the mixed vegetables with olive oil, salt, and pepper.
- On a baking sheet lined with parchment paper, arrange the vegetables.
- Drizzle the vegetables with balsamic vinegar.
- Roast the vegetables in the oven at 400°F (200°C) for 15-20 minutes or until tender.
- Serve the grilled salmon with roasted vegetables.

# Day 9:

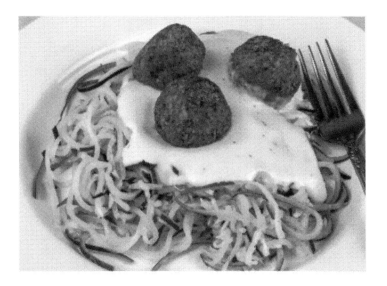

## Breakfast - Chocolate Banana Protein Smoothie

**Ingredients:**

- 1 ripe banana
- 1 scoop of chocolate protein powder
- 1 tablespoon almond butter
- 1 cup almond milk (unsweetened)
- 1 tablespoon cocoa powder
- 1 tablespoon honey (optional)
- Ice cubes

**Preparation:**

- In a blender, put all the ingredients and blend thoroughly until smooth.
- Add ice cubes for desired thickness.
- Serve chilled.

## Lunch - Quinoa and Avocado Salad

**Ingredients:**

- 1 cup cooked quinoa
- ½ avocado, diced
- ½ cup diced cucumber
- ½ cup cherry tomatoes, halved
- ¼ cup diced red onion
- 2 tablespoons chopped fresh cilantro
- Juice of 1 lime
- 1 tablespoon extra-virgin olive oil
- Salt and pepper to taste

**Preparation:**

- In a large bowl, combine cooked quinoa, avocado, cucumber, cherry tomatoes, red onion, and cilantro.
- Whisk together lime juice, olive oil, salt, and pepper in a small bowl.
- Pour the dressing over the quinoa and avocado salad and toss to combine.

- Serve chilled.

## Dinner - Turkey Meatballs with Zucchini Noodles

**Ingredients:**

- ½ pound ground turkey
- ¼ cup whole wheat breadcrumbs
- 1 egg
- 2 tablespoons grated Parmesan cheese
- 2 tablespoons chopped fresh parsley
- 1 garlic clove, minced
- Salt and pepper to taste
- 2 zucchinis, spiralized
- 1 cup marinara sauce

**Preparation:**

- In a bowl, combine ground turkey, breadcrumbs, egg, Parmesan cheese, parsley, minced garlic, salt, and pepper.
- Form the mixture into meatballs.
- Over medium heat, in a large skillet, heat the olive oil.
- Add the meatballs to the skillet and cook until browned on all sides and cooked through.

- Set the meatballs aside after you remove from the skillet.
- In the same skillet, add the spiralized zucchini and sauté for 2-3 minutes until tender.
- Pour the marinara sauce over the zucchini noodles and heat until warm.
- Serve the turkey meatballs over the zucchini noodles with marinara sauce.
- Enjoy!

**Day 10:**

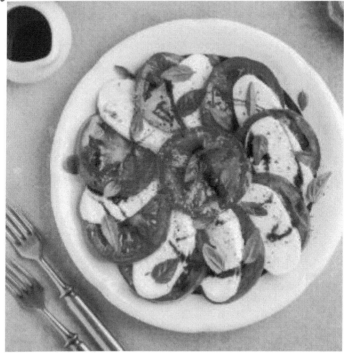

## Breakfast - Green Detox Smoothie
**Ingredients:**

- 1 cup spinach
- ½ cucumber, chopped
- 1 green apple, cored and chopped
- ½ ripe avocado
- Juice of 1 lemon
- 1 cup coconut water
- 1 tablespoon honey (optional)
- Ice cubes

**Preparation:**

In a blender, combine spinach, cucumber, green apple, avocado, lemon juice, coconut water, and honey (if desired).

Blend until smooth.

Add ice cubes for desired thickness.

Serve chilled.

## Lunch - Caprese Salad
**Ingredients:**

- 1 large tomato, sliced
- 4-6 fresh basil leaves
- 4 ounces fresh mozzarella cheese, sliced
- 1 tablespoon balsamic glaze

- 1 tablespoon extra-virgin olive oil
- Salt and pepper to taste

**Preparation:**

- Arrange tomato slices, basil leaves, and mozzarella cheese slices on a plate.
- Use the balsamic glaze and olive oil to drizzle the salad.
- Season with salt and pepper.
- Serve at room temperature.

## Dinner - Baked Cod with Quinoa and Steamed Broccoli

**Ingredients:**

- 1 cod fillet
- 1 tablespoon olive oil
- Juice of 1 lemon
- 1 teaspoon dried oregano
- Salt and pepper to taste
- 1 cup cooked quinoa
- Steamed broccoli florets

**Preparation:**

- Preheat the oven to 375°F (190°C).
- On a baking sheet lined with parchment paper, arrange the cod fillet.

- Use the olive oil and lemon juice to drizzle the cod.
- Sprinkle dried oregano, salt, and pepper over the cod.
- Bake the cod for 15-20 minutes or until it is thoroughly cooked.
- Serve the baked cod with cooked quinoa and steamed broccoli florets.
- Enjoy!

## Day 11:

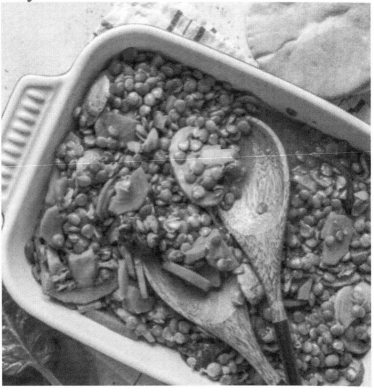

# Breakfast - Mixed Berry Overnight Oats

**Ingredients:**

- ½ cup rolled oats
- ½ cup almond milk (unsweetened)
- ¼ cup Greek yogurt
- 1 tablespoon chia seeds
- 1 tablespoon honey (optional)
- 1 cup straw-blue-raspberries
- 1 tablespoon crushed almonds

**Preparation:**

- In a jar or container, combine rolled oats, almond milk, Greek yogurt, chia seeds, and honey (if desired).
- Stir well to combine.
- Top with mixed berries and crushed almonds.
- Cover and refrigerate overnight.
- Serve chilled.

# Lunch - Spinach and Feta Stuffed Chicken Breast

**Ingredients:**

- 2 boneless, skinless chicken breasts
- 1 cup fresh spinach leaves
- ¼ cup crumbled feta cheese

- 1 garlic clove, minced
- Salt and pepper to taste
- 1 tablespoon olive oil

**Preparation:**

- Preheat the oven to 375°F (190°C).
- Slice a pocket in each chicken breast, being careful not to cut through completely.
- In a small bowl, combine spinach leaves, feta cheese, minced garlic, salt, and pepper.
- Fill the chicken breast pockets with a mixture of spinach and feta
- Over medium-high heat, in an oven-safe skillet, heat olive oil.
- Add the stuffed chicken breasts to the skillet and sear for 2-3 minutes on each side until browned.
- Move the skillet to the oven, and bake the chicken for 20 to 25 mins
- Serve hot.

## Dinner - Lentil Vegetable Curry
**Ingredients:**

- 1 cup cooked lentils
- 1 tablespoon olive oil
- 1 onion, diced

- 2 garlic cloves, minced
- 1 tablespoon curry powder
- 1 teaspoon ground cumin
- 1 teaspoon ground coriander
- 1 can diced tomatoes
- 1 cup vegetable broth
- 1 cup chopped vegetables (carrots, bell peppers, zucchini)
- Salt and pepper to taste
- Fresh cilantro for garnish

**Preparation:**

- Over medium heat in a large skillet, heat the olive oil
- Stir in the minced garlic and onion, and cook until softened.
- Stir in curry powder, ground cumin, and ground coriander, and cook for 1 minute.
- Add diced tomatoes (with juices) and vegetable broth to the skillet.
- Bring the mixture to a simmer.
- Stir in cooked lentils and chopped vegetables.
- Cover and cook for 15-20 minutes or until the vegetables are tender.

- Season with salt and pepper.
- Garnish with fresh cilantro.
- Serve with naan bread or rice, if desired.

**Day 12:**

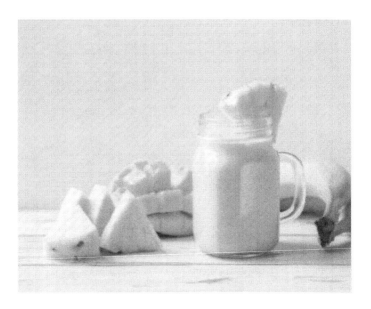

## Breakfast - Tropical Mango Smoothie
**Ingredients:**

- 1 cup frozen mango chunks
- ½ cup pineapple chunks
- 1 ripe banana
- ½ cup coconut milk (unsweetened)

- 1 tablespoon chia seeds
- 1 tablespoon honey (optional)
- Ice cubes

**Preparation:**

- In a blender, combine frozen mango chunks, pineapple chunks, ripe bananas, coconut milk, chia seeds, and honey (if desired).
- Blend until smooth.
- Add ice cubes for desired thickness.
- Serve chilled.

## Lunch - Quinoa and Black Bean Wrap
**Ingredients:**

- ½ cup cooked quinoa
- ½ cup black beans rinsed and drained
- ¼ cup diced bell peppers (any color)
- 2 tablespoons chopped fresh cilantro
- Juice of 1 lime
- Salt and pepper to taste
- Whole wheat tortillas
- Avocado slices (optional)

**Preparation:**

- In a bowl, combine cooked quinoa, black beans, diced bell peppers, chopped cilantro, lime juice, salt, and pepper.
- Warm the whole wheat tortillas.
- Place a scoop of the quinoa and black bean mixture onto each tortilla.
- Add avocado slices if desired.
- Tuck the sides of the tortillas in as you carefully roll them up.
- Serve the wraps cut in half.

# Dinner - Baked Eggplant Parmesan
**Ingredients:**

- 1 large eggplant, sliced into rounds
- Salt
- ½ cup whole wheat breadcrumbs
- ¼ cup grated Parmesan cheese
- 1 teaspoon dried oregano
- 1 teaspoon dried basil
- 1 cup marinara sauce
- ½ cup shredded mozzarella cheese
- Fresh basil leaves for garnish

**Preparation:**

- Place the eggplant slices in a colander and sprinkle salt over them. Let them sit for 30 minutes to draw out excess moisture.
- Preheat the oven to 375°F (190°C).
- Rinse the salt off the eggplant slices and pat them dry with paper towels.
- In a shallow bowl, combine breadcrumbs, grated Parmesan cheese, dried oregano, and dried basil.
- Coat both sides of each eggplant slice in the breadcrumb mixture.
- On a baking sheet with parchment paper, arrange the coated eggplant slices.
- Bake for 15-20 minutes or until the eggplant is tender and the breadcrumbs are golden.
- Remove the baking sheet from the oven and spoon marinara sauce over each eggplant slice.
- Use the shredded mozzarella cheese to sprinkle over the sauce.
- Return the baking sheet to the oven and bake for an additional 10 minutes or until the cheese is melted and bubbly.

- Garnish with fresh basil leaves.
- Serve hot.

## Day 13:

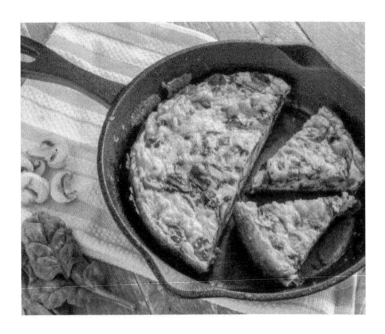

## Breakfast - Spinach and Mushroom Omelet
**Ingredients:**

- 3 large eggs
- 1 cup fresh spinach leaves
- ½ cup sliced mushrooms
- ¼ cup diced onion

- Salt and pepper to taste
- 1 teaspoon olive oil

**Preparation:**

- Whisk the eggs in a mixing dish until thoroughly combined. Set aside.
- Over medium heat in a non-stick skillet, heat olive oil.
- Add diced onion and sliced mushrooms to the skillet and sauté until softened.
- Add fresh spinach leaves to the skillet and cook until wilted.
- Over the vegetables in the skillet, pour the beaten eggs.
- Season with salt and pepper.
- Cook until the edges of the omelet are set.
- Gently lift the edges with a spatula and tilt the skillet to allow the uncooked eggs to flow underneath.
- Continue cooking until the omelet is fully set but still slightly moist on top.
- The omelet should be folded in half and placed on a plate.
- Serve hot.

## Lunch - Greek Salad with Grilled Chicken

**Ingredients:**

- 4 ounces grilled chicken breast, sliced
- 2 cups mixed greens
- ¼ cup sliced cucumber
- ¼ cup cherry tomatoes, halved
- 2 tablespoons sliced Kalamata olives
- 2 tablespoons crumbled feta cheese
- Juice of 1 lemon
- 1 tablespoon extra-virgin olive oil
- Salt and pepper to taste

**Preparation:**

- In a large bowl, combine mixed greens, sliced cucumber, cherry tomatoes, Kalamata olives, and crumbled feta cheese.
- Top with sliced grilled chicken.
- Whisk the lemon juice, olive oil, salt, and pepper in a small bowl.
- Drizzle the dressing over the salad.
- Toss to combine.
- Serve chilled.

# Dinner - Baked Turkey Breast with Roasted Vegetables

**Ingredients:**

- 1 turkey breast, bone-in, skin-on
- 1 tablespoon olive oil
- 1 teaspoon dried thyme
- 1 teaspoon dried rosemary
- Salt and pepper to taste
- 2 cups mixed vegetables (carrots, Brussels sprouts, sweet potatoes)
- 1 tablespoon balsamic vinegar

**Preparation:**

- Preheat the oven to 375°F (190°C).
- Place the turkey breast on a baking sheet lined with parchment paper.
- Rub the turkey breast with olive oil, dried thyme, dried rosemary, salt, and pepper.
- Bake for 1 to 1.5 hours or until the internal temperature reaches 165°F (74°C).
- In the meantime, toss the mixed vegetables with olive oil, salt, and pepper.
- Place the vegetables on a separate baking sheet lined with parchment paper.

- Drizzle the vegetables with balsamic vinegar.
- Roast the vegetables in the oven at 400°F (200°C) for 25-30 minutes or until tender.
- Serve the baked turkey breast with roasted vegetables.
- Enjoy!

## Day 14:

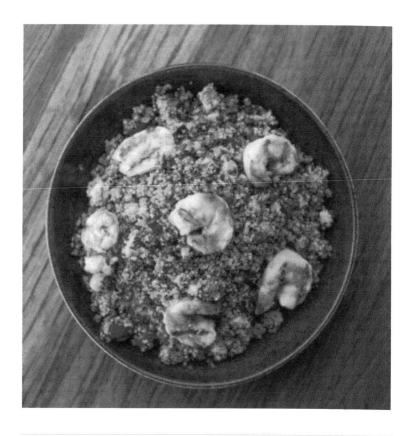

# Breakfast - Berry Chia Seed Pudding

**Ingredients:**

- ¼ cup chia seeds
- 1 cup almond milk (unsweetened)
- 1 tablespoon honey or maple syrup
- ½ teaspoon vanilla extract
- 1 cup straw-blue-raspberries
- 1 tablespoon shredded coconut (optional)

**Preparation:**

- • Mix the chia seeds, almond milk, honey or maple syrup, and vanilla extract in a bowl.
- • Be sure to stir thoroughly to spread the chia seeds evenly.
- • Place the bowl in the refrigerator for at least 4 hours or overnight.
- When ready to serve, give the chia seed mixture a good stir to break up any clumps.
- Layer the chia seed pudding with mixed berries in a glass or jar.
- Top with shredded coconut if desired.
- Serve chilled.

## Lunch - Quinoa Salad with Grilled Shrimp

**Ingredients:**

- ½ cup cooked quinoa
- 4 ounces grilled shrimp
- 1 cup mixed greens
- ¼ cup diced cucumber
- ¼ cup diced bell peppers (any color)
- 2 tablespoons chopped fresh parsley
- Juice of 1 lemon
- 1 tablespoon extra-virgin olive oil
- Salt and pepper to taste

**Preparation:**

- In a bowl, combine cooked quinoa, grilled shrimp, mixed greens, diced cucumber, diced bell peppers, and chopped parsley.
- Whisk the lemon juice, olive oil, salt, and pepper in a small bowl.
- Drizzle the dressing over the quinoa salad.
- Toss to combine.
- Serve chilled.

# Dinner - Quinoa with Asparagus and Baked Salmon

**Ingredients:**

- 1 salmon fillet
- 1 tablespoon olive oil
- Juice of 1 lemon
- 1 teaspoon dried dill
- Salt and pepper to taste
- 1 bunch asparagus, trimmed
- 1 cup cooked quinoa

**Preparation:**

- Preheat the oven to 375°F (190°C).
- On a baking sheet lined with parchment paper, arrange the salmon fillet.
- Drizzle the salmon with olive oil and lemon juice.
- Sprinkle dried dill, salt, and pepper over the salmon.
- Arrange trimmed asparagus around the salmon on the baking sheet.
- Bake the salmon for 12 to 15 mins, or until it flakes easily.
- While the salmon is baking, heat the cooked quinoa.
- Serve the baked salmon with asparagus and quinoa.
- Enjoy!

# Day 15:

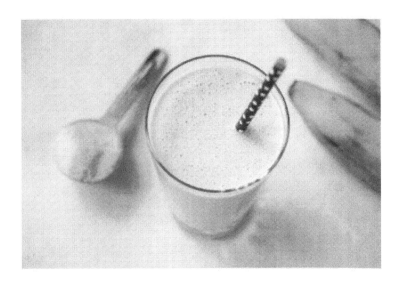

## Breakfast - Almond Butter Banana Smoothie
**Ingredients:**

- 1 ripe banana
- 2 tablespoons almond butter
- 1 cup almond milk (unsweetened)
- 1 tablespoon honey or maple syrup
- Ice cubes

**Preparation:**

- In a blender, combine ripe banana, almond butter, almond milk, and honey or maple syrup.
- Blend until smooth.
- Add ice cubes for desired thickness.
- Serve chilled.

# Lunch - Mediterranean Hummus Wrap
**Ingredients:**

- Whole wheat wrap or tortilla
- ¼ cup hummus
- ¼ cup sliced cucumber
- ¼ cup sliced tomatoes
- 2 tablespoons sliced Kalamata olives
- 2 tablespoons crumbled feta cheese
- Fresh spinach leaves

**Preparation:**

- Spread hummus evenly on the whole wheat wrap or tortilla.
- Layer sliced cucumber, sliced tomatoes, Kalamata olives, crumbled feta cheese, and fresh spinach leaves on top of the hummus.

- Roll up the wrap tightly.
- Serve the wrap in half.

## Dinner - Grilled Chicken with Quinoa and Steamed Vegetables

**Ingredients:**

- 4 ounces grilled chicken breast
- 1 cup cooked quinoa
- Assorted steamed vegetables (broccoli, cauliflower, carrots)
- Lemon wedges for serving

**Preparation:**

- Season the grilled chicken breast with your choice of herbs and spices.
- Grill the chicken until cooked through.
- Slice the grilled chicken into strips.
- Serve the grilled chicken with cooked quinoa and steamed vegetables.
- Squeeze fresh lemon juice over the chicken and vegetables before serving.
- Enjoy!

# TROUBLESHOOTING THE WHOLE BODY RESET

**Review the Program Guidelines:** Start by carefully reviewing the guidelines and instructions provided by the Whole Body Reset program. Ensure you understand the program's principles, recommended foods, portion sizes, and any restrictions or modifications specific to seniors.

**Consult with a Healthcare Professional:** Before starting any weight loss program, it's crucial to consult with your healthcare professional, especially if you're over 50. They can assess your overall health, review any medical conditions or medications that may impact your weight loss journey, and provide personalized advice.

**Evaluate Your Calorie Intake:** Check if you're consuming an appropriate number of calories. As we age, our metabolic rate tends to slow down. Therefore, you may need to adjust your calorie intake to account for this change. Ensure you're neither consuming too few calories, which can be detrimental to your health, nor exceeding your calorie needs, which may hinder weight loss progress.

**Monitor Portion Sizes:** Pay attention to your portion sizes. Seniors often have different nutritional requirements, so it's crucial to consume balanced meals with appropriate portions of protein, carbohydrates, and healthy fats. Use measuring cups, a food scale, or visual cues to ensure you're not overeating or underestimating your portions.

**Increase Physical Activity:** Regular physical activity is vital for weight loss and overall health. If you're not already active, consider incorporating moderate aerobic exercises like walking, or swimming into your routine. Strength training exercises, with proper guidance from a professional, can help preserve muscle mass and improve metabolism.

**Address Emotional and Stress Eating:** Emotional and stress eating can hinder weight loss progress. Pay attention to your eating habits and identify any triggers that lead to excessive or mindless eating. Find alternative coping mechanisms such as engaging in hobbies, practicing mindfulness or meditation, or seeking support from friends, family, or a counselor.

**Stay Hydrated:** Proper hydration is essential for overall health and weight management. Ensure you're drinking enough water throughout the day. Water can help curb appetite, support digestion, and prevent dehydration-related issues that can affect metabolism and energy levels.

**Track Progress:** Keep a record of your food intake, exercise routine, and any challenges or successes you encounter. Use a journal, mobile app, or online tools to track your progress. This can help identify patterns, areas of improvement, or potential issues that may require troubleshooting.

**Seek Support:** Consider joining a support group, finding a workout buddy, or partnering with a friend or family member who shares similar goals. Having someone to share your experiences, challenges, and successes can provide motivation and accountability.

**Patience and Persistence:** Remember that weight loss takes time and effort, especially for seniors. Be patient with yourself, stay committed to your goals, and celebrate every small milestone along the way. Don't give up if you experience setbacks or plateaus. Instead, use them as opportunities to reevaluate your approach, make necessary adjustments, and keep moving forward.

Remember, the Whole Body Reset weight loss program may not be suitable for everyone, especially those with underlying health conditions.

Always prioritize your safety and consult with a healthcare professional before making any significant changes to your diet or exercise routine.

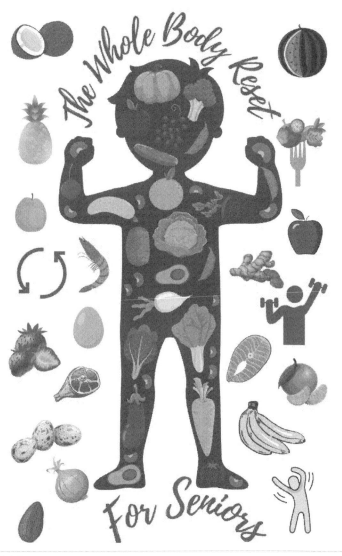

# CONCLUSION

In conclusion, the Whole Body Reset weight loss program offers a comprehensive and effective approach for seniors who are looking to achieve their weight loss goals. This program recognizes the unique needs and challenges that seniors face when it comes to weight management and focuses on addressing them with a holistic approach.

One of the key strengths of the Whole Body Reset program is its emphasis on overall health and well-being. It doesn't solely focus on weight loss but also prioritizes improving seniors' overall physical fitness, mental well-being, and lifestyle habits. By incorporating a combination of balanced nutrition, regular exercise, and mindfulness techniques, the program promotes sustainable weight loss and long-term health benefits.

Additionally, the Whole Body Reset program takes into account the specific nutritional requirements of seniors. It provides personalized meal plans and guidance to ensure that seniors receive the necessary nutrients while maintaining a calorie deficit for weight loss. This approach helps prevent muscle loss and promotes healthy aging.

Furthermore, the program encourages regular physical activity tailored to the capabilities and limitations of seniors. It includes a variety of exercises that help improve strength, endurance, and balance. These exercises not only contribute to weight loss but also support joint health and reduce the risk of age-related conditions.

The Whole Body Reset program also emphasizes the importance of mindset and stress management. It incorporates mindfulness practices, such as meditation and relaxation techniques, to help seniors develop a positive relationship with food, manage emotional eating, and reduce stress levels. This holistic approach promotes sustainable lifestyle changes and long-term weight management.

Made in the USA
Las Vegas, NV
07 January 2024

84043626R10048